YOUR GUIDE TO BREAST SURGERY

Dr Laith Barnouti, FRACS (Plastic)
Specialist Plastic Surgeon

For further information contact:
Dr Laith Barnouti, Specialist Plastic Surgeon
Tel: 1 300 002 006; +61 2 9561 0222
Address: 2/37 Bay St Glebe NSW 2037 Australia
http://www.plasticsurgery-sydney.com.au
Email: drbarnouti@australiaplasticsurgery.com.au

Medical Editor: Tina Allen (www.tinaallen.com.au)

Book and Cover Design: Phoenix Spencer Publishing

Graphic Design: Kaarina Allen

A catalogue record for this book is available from the National Library of Australia.

TABLE OF CONTENTS

AUTHOR'S NOTE

This book marks more than 20 years since I started my surgical training at the Queen Elizabeth Hospital in South Australia and more than 15 years of practising in the field of plastic surgery.

In 2008, I was granted my fellowship of the Royal Australasian College of Surgeons, FRACS (Plastic).

In 2020, I was invited to become a Conjoint Lecturer in medicine and surgery at the University of New South Wales and from July 2022 I have been a Conjoint Senior Lecturer.

I have travelled the world seeking more knowledge, answers and experience in plastic surgery. My international fellowship training was in Rio De Janeiro (Brazil), Stockholm (Sweden) and Gent (Belgium). I feel privileged to have trained with some of the best surgeons in the world. It opened my mind and widened my knowledge.

These last 15 years plus of running plastic surgery clinics in Sydney hold an excellent record of safety. I provide my patients with the best possible care and aesthetic outcomes. This includes delivering surgery in a meticulous manner and not ignoring the vital post-operative and recovery phases.

I am also very open and honest with patients. Every week, I send patients away; telling them they don't need surgery.

Patients are often surprised when they are told by a specialist plastic surgeon that surgery is not recommended for them. Surgery needs to be performed for the right reasons. I remind patients every day that surgery is trauma to the body in a controlled manner.

I am not in the business of "selling surgery". Rather I pride myself in providing the best health advice to my patients and putting their health first and foremost. As a medical practitioner, I have taken the Hippocratic Oath to "do no harm".

While plastic surgery can be very satisfying by bringing happiness to patients and changing their lives, I take this profession very seriously. I hold a great deal of responsibility because patients trust me with their health.

This is done through careful consultation and communication. Planning for surgery will only be put in place if I feel it is in the patient's best interests.

Finally, it's important to mention that all the "before and after" photos in this book are of patients who I have operated on during the last 15 years. None have been altered or Photoshopped.

Enjoy the book.

Dr Laith Barnouti

Specialist Plastic Surgeon, fracs
Conjoint Senior Lecturer, University of NSW
Sydney, Australia
August 2024

ACKNOWLEDGMENTS

Many thanks to my beautiful and original wife, Dr Zoe Potres and my three amazing children Lara, Lydia and Oscar. You keep me grounded.

I would like to acknowledge the support of my energetic and enthusiastic father, Dr Ramzi Barnouti OAM and my mother, Hannah, who is always keen to know what I am doing and if I am busy enough with my work!

I am grateful to have been brought up as a member of the medical "Barnouti" family who emphasise achievements, hard work and ethics. They have provided me with guidance, love and support along the way.

With a special mention to my mentors in the plastic surgery field: Dr Patrick Tonnard (Belgium), Dr Per Heden (Sweden), the late Professor Ivo Pitanguy (Brazil), Dr Alex Verpaele (Belgium), Dr Daniel Baker (USA), Dr Michael Poole (Australia), Dr Michael Baldwin (Australia), Dr David Pennington (Australia) and Dr Paul Curtin (Australia).

I consider myself lucky to have worked with some of the best surgeons in the world and learned their techniques, ethics and commitment to work.

I would like to thank my work partner and skilled surgeon, Dr Mark Kohout, for a great working relationship throughout the years. We run and manage one of the most successful plastic surgery clinics in Australia. It is a partnership that is based on trust and respect. We share not only knowledge and ideas, but also great responsibilities in always attempting to deliver the best standard of care and aesthetic outcomes for our patients.

A successful practice requires mature, dedicated and committed staff. I have been lucky enough to have worked with great anaesthetists, surgical assistants, registrars and nurses. All made possible by an exceptional personal assistant, Jessie Elliot. Thank you.

I would like to acknowledge the staff at Westmead Private, Hunters Hill Private, City West Specialist and Sydney Private hospitals for providing a safe environment and great facilities for my patients.

And finally, to my patients who keep me intellectually motivated by seeking answers to different problems… this book is for you.

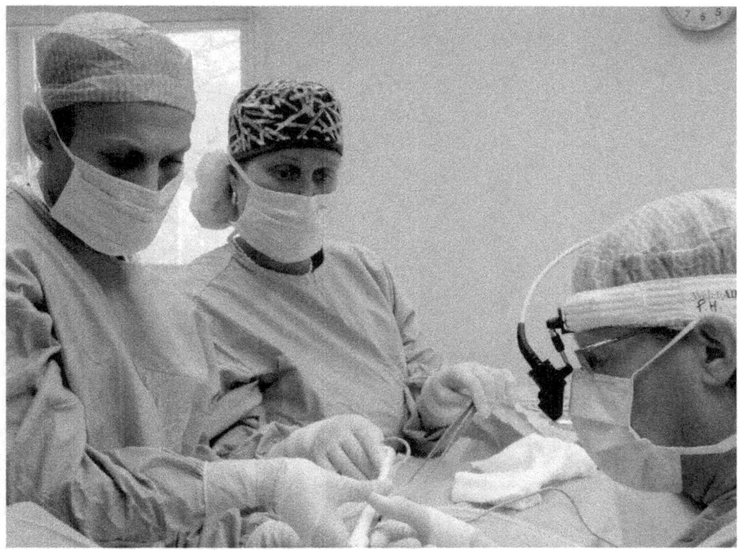

Dr Laith Barnouti at Akademikliniken Plastikkirurgi – Sweden's largest plastic surgery clinic – performing breast surgery with Dr Per Heden. Dr Barnouti spent three months in Stockholm, Sweden perfecting his skills in breast surgery.

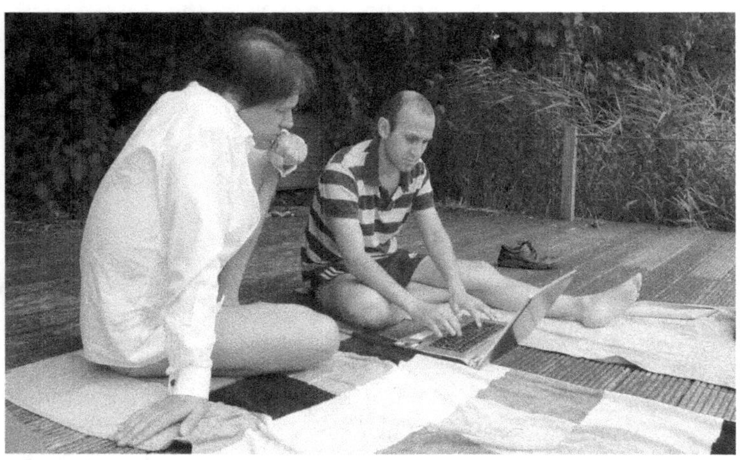

Here is a view into my private life as I write a plastic surgery paper with Dr Patrick Tonnard next to a private lake in Gent, Belgium.

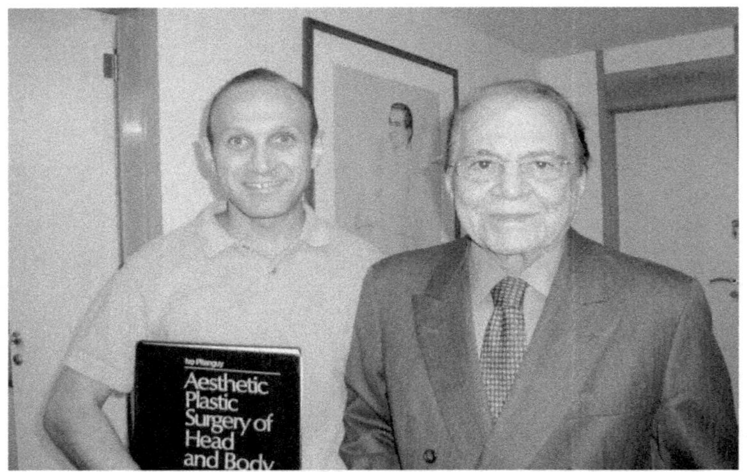

Dr Laith Barnouti in Rio De Janeiro with the father of modern plastic surgery, Professor Ivo Pitanguy. "I feel privileged to have worked and learned from the Master of the trade," says Dr Barnouti of Prof Pitanguy who died in 2016.

INTRODUCTION

Over my 15 years of practicing as a specialist plastic surgeon, I have heard stories from many patients about their dissatisfaction with their breasts or other parts of their body. This ranges from staring into the mirror and lifting their breasts higher, to not feeling confident going to the beach in a swimsuit or bikini.

Before reading this book, ask yourself the following questions:

Have you ever felt sub-conscious about the appearance of your breasts?

Were you born with a flat chest of asymmetrical breasts?

Has your breast shape changed after having children?

Do you feel that pregnancy or weight fluctuation may have affected your breasts? Does this make you feel less attractive and less confident?

Have you ever wondered if you could turn back the hands of time?

If you answered yes to any of the above questions, then this book is for you.

How we feel about our bodies and physical appearance can have a huge impact on our confidence and general wellbeing. For example, disliking your breasts and body can have a negative impact on our relationships with other people.

Unfortunately, there is very little you can do personally to change your breasts or a part of the body you were born with – or how it changes as you age and are exposed to physiological or pathological changes.

You may have wrestled with the notion of having plastic surgery but are still not sure. You don't want to end up looking like one of those over-the-top plastic surgery disasters, who have achieved the opposite of the desired effect by drawing attention to their age. But at the same time, you may see or know people who you admire for the successful "work" they have had done on their breasts or body, because they look younger and more vibrant than they did before.

It's no secret that plastic surgery can help you achieve what you want for your breasts and body.

So, if you want the confidence that comes from looking your best, then this book is for you. It focusses on the positive change in your appearance that can be achieved safely by plastic surgery when performed by expert hands.

This book will also answer many of the questions asked by women who are considering breast surgery, including how to choose a surgeon and what are the recovery times post-surgery.

Your Guide to Breast Surgery follows the publication of Dr Barnouti's first book, *Your Guide to Modern Plastic Surgery.* As the title of his previous book suggests, Dr Barnouti uses the most up-to-date surgical and non-surgical procedures in his practice. This includes performing minimally invasive breast enlargement surgery through a small scar in the areolar line around the nipple, as opposed to an incision in the breast crease.

Breast size and shape are often a big concern for women and can cause serious confidence issues. Breast surgery is one of our most frequently requested plastic surgery procedures because breast changes are common due to developmental reasons, hormonal changes, weight fluctuation, pregnancy or breastfeeding.

Whether you are interested in breast reduction, enlargement, lift or removal and replacement of an old implant, the best advice is for your breast size and shape to be in proportion to your body habitus. That means that the width, height and projection of your breasts has to fit within the boundaries of your chest and remain in harmony with the width of your shoulders and hips. Our aim is to provide natural results for all of these procedures.

Sometimes breast surgery is combined with other surgical procedures. Post pregnancy body restorative surgery, which is often referred to as a 'Mummy Makeover', includes breast enlargement, a breast lift with or without implants, or breast reduction.

Breast surgery can also be a component of post weight-loss surgery. Extra skin, fat and weak muscles around the abdomen and hips can be caused naturally by pregnancy, the ageing process or stress-related weight gain that proves resistant to an improved diet and exercise. Known as "stubborn fat areas", they may be hard to shift through exercise and diet alone. Many patients opt for a tummy tuck, which is sometimes called abdominoplasty, and breast surgery because they want to wear a wider variety of clothing and improve their personal body image.

If you want to be in the safest possible hands, then make sure that you do your homework and choose a specialist plastic surgeon, a specialist aneasthetist and a fully accredited hospital for your surgery. In the case of the specialist plastic surgeon, look for the letters FRACS (Plastic), or the equivalent qualification from an overseas college of surgeons, after their name.

Either myself, or your own specialist plastic surgeon, will explain the wide range of surgical and non-surgical options available to you, what realistic results you can hope to achieve and ultimately, how your life can be drastically changed.

My patients range in age from 18 to 75, but most are in their forties and fifties. While I do preform breast surgery on men, this book is mainly concerned with surgery for women.

Your age and the type of procedure you choose will influence the length of your recovery time. However, you should plan for six weeks for a full recovery, during which you dedicate time to taking things quietly and attending post-surgery consultations for dressing changes and wound care. Most patients can return to light office-based work after two weeks.

The good news is that the surgical and non-surgical options highlighted in this book are no longer the exclusive domain of celebrities. Plastic surgery has become more affordable over the years because of the increased number of surgical options and providers as well as the availability of payment plan options.

Prior to making any decisions about whether to have plastic surgery, it is important to consider all the alternatives. Your specialist plastic surgeon will outline any possible risks of undergoing surgery and provide advice as to whether cosmetic surgery is for you or not. It is advisable to take your time and discuss your decision with someone you can trust.

It is also worth mentioning that the cultural shift in this age of social media can sometimes force people to become "too obsessed" with their appearance. While cosmetic surgery can improve and enhance your breasts and body, a "perfect outcome" is both unrealistic and unachievable.

If you're looking for "perfection", remember that perfection is unattainable. The human body is naturally asymmetrical, and it can be even more beautiful for its asymmetry.

I remind patients that surgery has limitations and that some surgical procedures may not be in their best interests. However, usually there are real solutions available that will rejuvenate and improve your looks as well as boosting your confidence.

CHAPTER ONE

Breast Enlargement

Breast enlargement, which is sometimes called breast augmentation, is among the most common procedures I perform and worldwide it is one of the most popular procedures for women. Many women desire a curvier figure. In fact, studies have shown that more than 50 per cent of women wish to alter the appearance of their breasts.

Breast size is a matter of personal choice; however, the modern ideal of female beauty and femininity places an emphasis on breasts that are aesthetically pleasing in all states of dress and undress.

My patients choose to have breast enlargements for six main reasons:

1) To increase the size of their breasts;

2) Because their breast shape has been compromised by pregnancy or ageing due to inflating-deflating phenomena, fat atrophy or gravitational forces;

3) To correct congenital or developmental breast problems which have resulted in smaller breasts;

4) Because their breasts are not symmetrical in size and/or shape;

5) Because their breasts have been removed as a result of breast cancer; or

6) Because of breast injuries, such as scars or burns, that have limited their breast growth.

Deciding to go ahead with breast augmentation is a very personal decision which should not be made casually or lightly. I have no hesitation in advising some patients that they do not need the surgery and to save their time, money and effort if I do not feel the surgery is in their best interest. This is especially the case for those women who have good breast volume or are still in their childbearing/breastfeeding years.

Everyone's body is different, and everyone has a different vision of the ideal. There is no one ideal. The shape, texture, profile, width, height and volume of breast augmentation will depend on the patient's body type, desires and lifestyle. There is no "one size fits all" approach and every woman has her own reasons for considering breast enlargement.

The surgeon's experience and vision play a significant role in guiding the patient to what is best for them. I do highly recommend to patients that three objectives need to be met with breast surgery:

1) longevity of maintaining perky breasts;

2) aesthetics (appearance) of the breasts; and

3) practicality.

It should be remembered that too-large breasts can cause neck/shoulder pain, they will drop more quickly and they have shorter longevity, i.e. the benefits of the procedure will be more short-lived.

Breast enlargement can be achieved through fat injection and/or implant surgery.

1.1 Breast Enlargement Using Fat Injections

This is a minimally invasive procedure as it uses fat that has been removed by liposuction from other parts of your body. I then purify the fatty cells and inject them into your breasts.

Fat transfer breast enlargement is not new; however, the low survival of the transplanted fat cells has previously been a limiting factor. This procedure has seen a resurgence in recent years due to an improved fat survival technique and the fact that it is minimally invasive.

It is a great option for women who are looking for a relatively small increase in breast size and would prefer natural results. I routinely use fat transfer when the patient wants her breasts to be enlarged by only one cup size. I also use this technique if the patient has implant rippling, as it is a great way to cover the edges of the implants and enhance the shape.

Another good indication for breast enlargement by fat injection is when the patient wants to replace their existing implants with larger ones, but their chest anatomy does not allow for a larger prosthesis. Fat injections will give them further enhancement. In these scenarios, a single stage procedure will usually suffice.

If the patient wishes to have a larger increase in her breast size by fat injection, i.e. two-to-three cup sizes bigger, then such an outcome can only be achieved by using a multistage procedure. The fat transfer needs to be performed two-to-three times, six months apart as some of the fat that is injected will be absorbed and/or disappear.

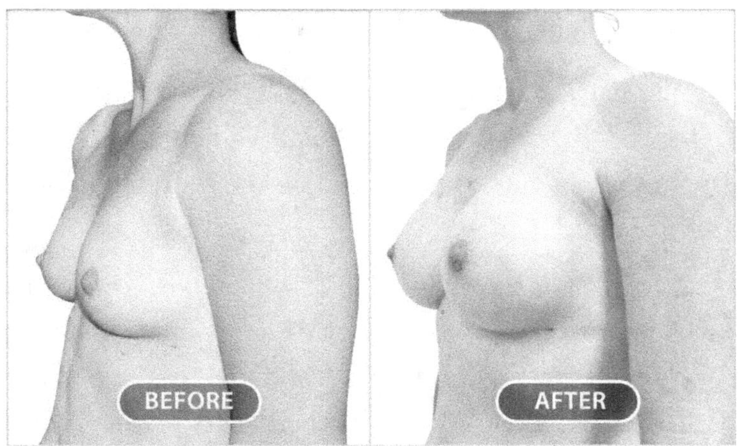

Breast augmentation with 240cc round breast implants. Note the perfect nipple position and proportionate chest.

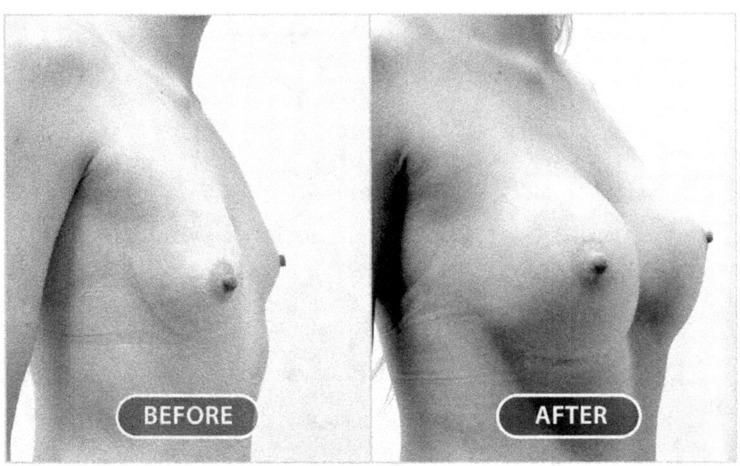

Breast augmentation with 300cc round breast implants. Natural outcome.

1.2 Breast Enlargement Using Implants

The alternative to fat injections is breast enlargement using implants. If the decision to go ahead with implant surgery is reached, then it is vital to choose the right technique, approach and implant.

Silicone implants made in the USA and Europe generally have lifetime guarantees against rupture and/or leakage. Silicone implants are the gold standard. They are made from a rubber shell filled with a highly cohesive silicone gel, which makes them lighter, softer and offers a more natural feel than saline implants.

I avoid using saline implants, due to their propensity for leakage, their unnatural feel and their generally suboptimal results.

Next, we consider the shape of the implants:

- Traditional round breast implants can be either smooth or textured. For under-the-muscle breast enlargements, there is no statistically significant difference between using smooth or textured breast implants. However, for above-the-muscle breast enlargement, textured round or teardrop implants (see below) are best.

- Teardrop breast implants produce a very natural breast shape and are also known as natural implants or anatomical breast implants. Teardrop implants are only made in a coarse texture. The Therapeutic

Goods Administration (TGA) in Australia suspended some of these implants in 2019 due to their link with Anaplastic Large Cell Lymphoma (ALCL). This will be discussed in the following section: Breast Implant Removal & Replacement Surgery.

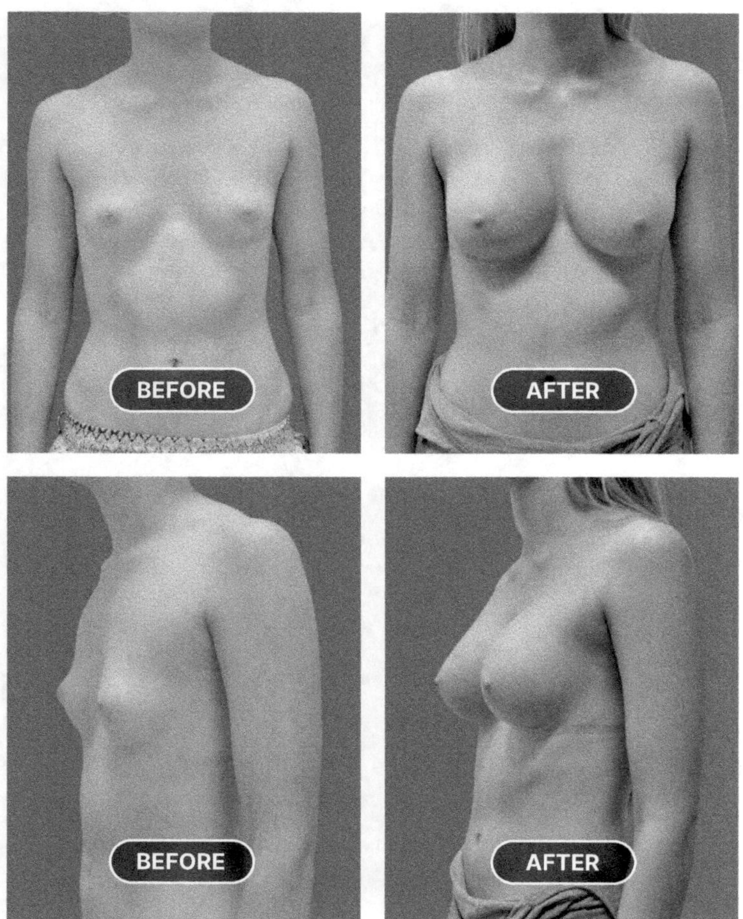

Breast augmentation using 320 cc round implants showing nice breast symmetry, cleavage and upper pole fullness in the after photos.

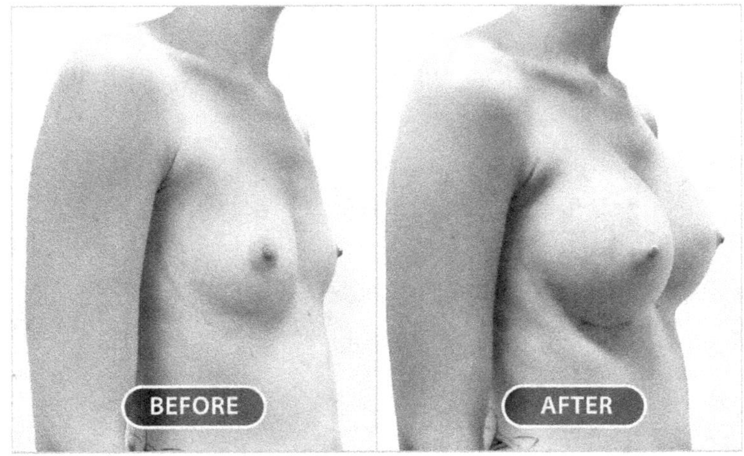

Breast augmentation with 350cc round implants; dual plane.

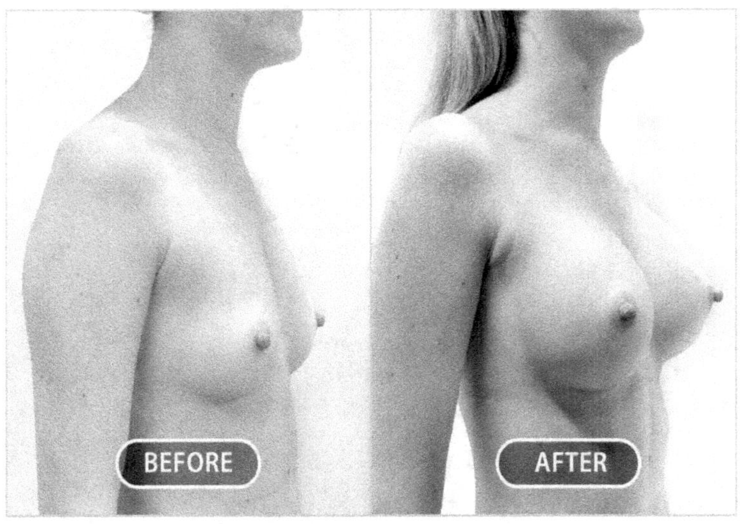

Breast augmentation with 360cc round breast implants; dual plane.

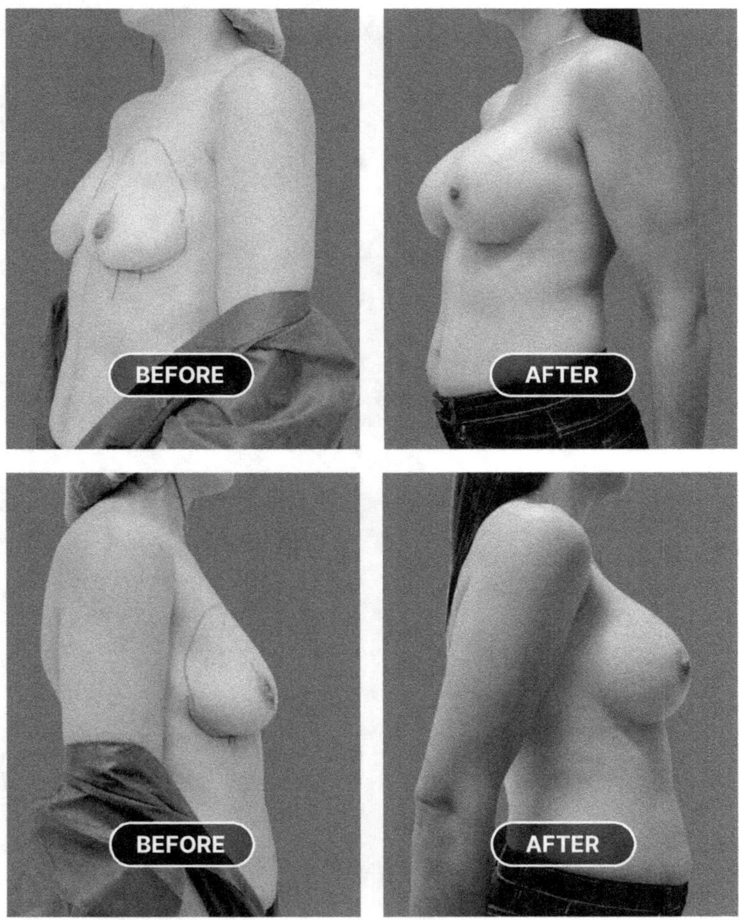

Breast augmentation with 360 cc round nano textured breast implants: dual plane. The procedure was performed through a small incision in the lower part of the areolar. This produces the best quality scar, which is literally invisible six months post-surgery for women with dark or Asian skin.

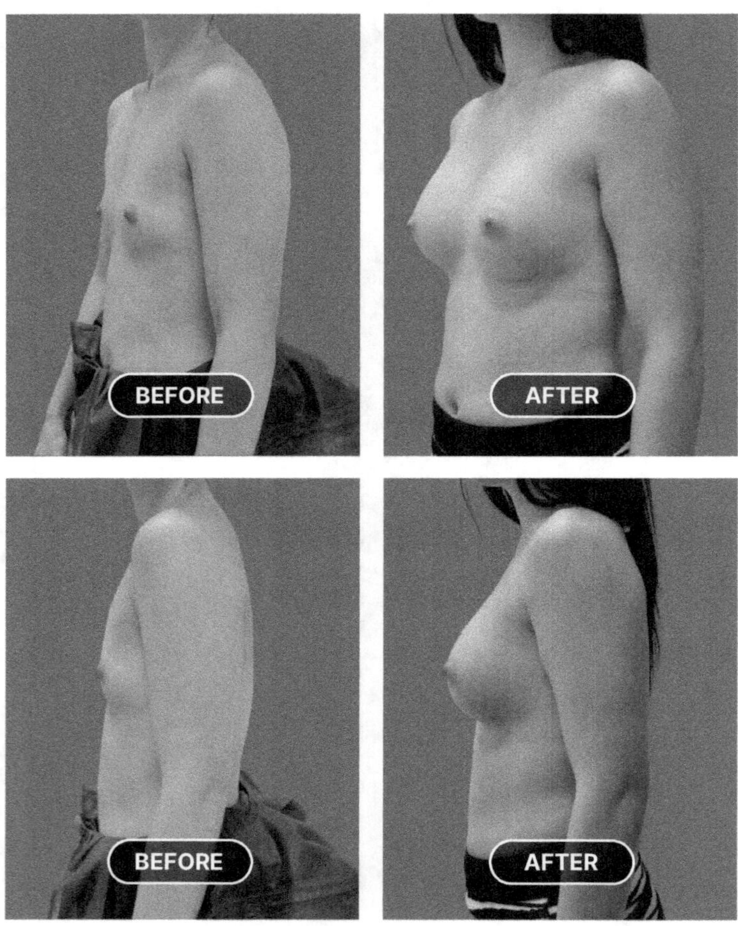

Breast augmentation with 320 cc round breast implants: dual submuscular plane. The upper pole deformity in the before photo has been corrected by the implant which sits under the pectoralis muscle and pushes out the breast tissue. The result is natural looking breasts.

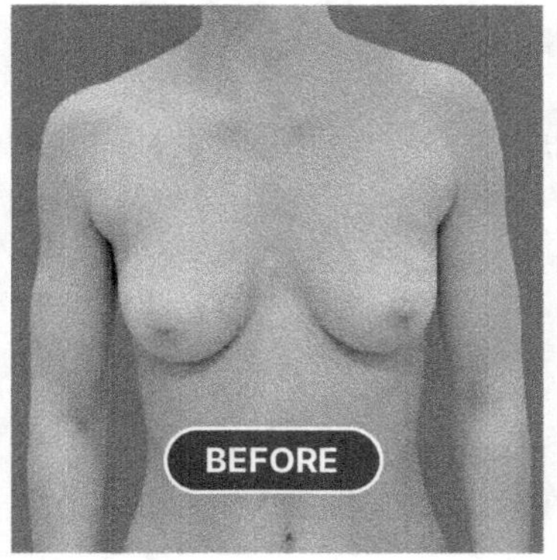

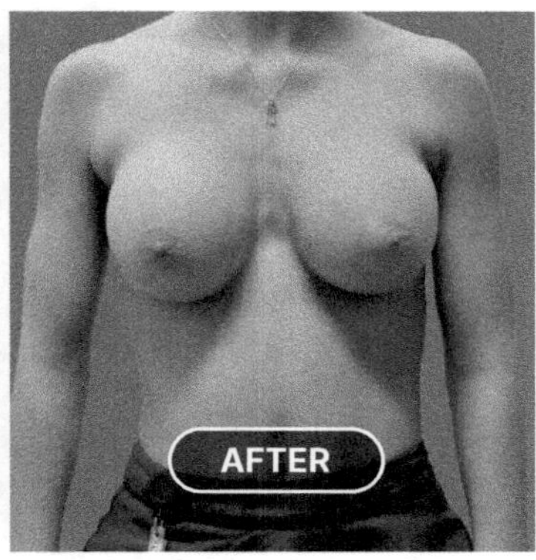

Breast augmentation with 290 cc extra high silicone implants.

Safe Breast Implants Surgery Technique

Upon making these decisions, the next step is the surgery. It's absolutely vital that the following steps of the "Safe Breast Implants Surgery Technique" are followed by your specialist plastic surgeon to optimise outcomes and minimise complications:

1) The patient is to have a shower the night before or the morning of the surgery.

2) When the patient is under general anaesthetic and before skin preparation with Betadine, scrub the patient's skin/chest/breast with a Betadine scrub.

3) Then perform routine Betadine preparation and draping.

4) Use intravenous antibiotic prophylaxis 20 minutes before the surgical incision, and two additional doses after surgery and prior to patient's discharge.

5) Use nipple shields to prevent spillage of bacteria into the pocket.

6) Use new instruments in deep planes, that were not used on the skin.

7) Perform a careful dissection.

8) Avoid unnecessary dissection into the breast tissue because this is traumatic and increases patient recovery time.

9) Be careful to maintain haemostasis in order to prevent and stop bleeding.

10) Change surgical gloves repeatedly as you get underneath the muscle. This will prevent skin contamination deep under the muscle pocket.

11) Use the "No Touch" Technique, as well as another change of gloves prior to handling the implants.

12) Use a dual-plane technique, when required.

13) Perform pocket irrigation with correct proven triple antibiotic solution, saline, Betadine or a combination of these solutions.

14) Minimise the length of time during opening, repositioning and replacement of the implant.

15) Prevent friction between the implant and skin, which can contaminate the implant. Friction is avoided by using a protective funnel to guide the implant

into the cavity and protect any contact between the skin and the implant.

16) Use a small drain, which is left in place for only 3–4 hours after surgery. It is important that the pocket is absolutely dry prior to the patient going home. The drain will empty the residual fluid/ blood/wash solution from the pocket.

17) Close the cavity in layers, leaving the suture knots away from the implants.

18) Use a closure with deep tissue and dermal eversion technique, especially with the breast crease incision, to ensure minimal scarring.

19) Seal the wound with fine dissolving sutures and do not leave any palpable suture knot directly under the skin surface.

20) Secure the wound with an additional protective glue barrier.

Such careful execution delivers the best outcomes as well as minimising the post-operative risks and long-term complications.

Such procedures should only be performed by an experienced specialist plastic surgeon. This will ensure the best possible outcome so that the breast augmentation meets the patient's needs, revision surgery is avoided and the procedure doesn't look like an obvious "boob job".

An excellent breast augmentation looks natural, with a gentle sloping off the chest wall to natural fullness, natural cleavage without webbing between the breasts, and a certain amount of perkiness. It lasts for about ten years without long-term issues such as rippling, neck pain double bubble or bottoming out.

Breast augmentation is a 60–90 minute procedure that, when performed correctly, can dramatically alter the way a woman feels about her body.

For women who want to maintain their current size or have larger breast volume and are currently experiencing sagginess in their breast tissue, breast augmentation can be performed at the same time as breast lift surgery.

1.3 Breast Implant Removal & Replacement Surgery

Breast implant removal surgery is performed under general anaesthesia and takes approximately two hours. It is usually performed as day surgery.

The three most common breast implant removal surgery techniques are:

1. Breast implant removal with capsulectomy – incisions will be made in the same place as the breast implant surgery was performed. A part or full section of the capsule surrounding the implants will be removed and sent for histopathological examination.

2. Breast implant removal and replacement with capsulectomy – as above with insertion of a new set of implants. Usually patients request higher projecting and slightly larger implants.

3. Breast implant removal with breast lift – some patients require a breast lift when they have their breast implants removed or replaced with smaller ones. The surgery is designed to remove the excess breast skin and tighten the breast tissue to provide better support. The areolas are often re-sized to better fit the new shape of the woman's breasts.

Whilst recovery from breast implant surgery varies from person to person, it is usually smoother than the initial breast implant surgery. However, if you have a breast lift after your breast implants have been removed, your breasts will feel tight for a few weeks.

Most women are able to return to work five days after surgery and experience minimal discomfort. If you've had breast implants removed due to capsular contracture, there will be more discomfort and the recovery time will be longer.

Breast implant removal scars typically heal very well and are often inconspicuous. It is important to note that they heal in stages with the process taking three-to-four months.

You will need to avoid lifting anything over five kilograms (11 pounds) or exercising excessively for the first six weeks after your surgery. While you will usually be able to resume normal activity after six weeks, your breasts will take three-to-six months to settle into their new position.

When a highly trained and experienced plastic surgeon performs breast implant removal/replacement surgery, the complications and risks will be minimal. However, it is important to note that the risks and complications can include:

- Blood collection or what is known as haematoma;

- Infection, which may necessitate the removal of the implants;

- Development of thick, red and painful scars, which may last for a few years;

- Numbness of the breast and/or nipples; and

- Breast deformity or sagging of the breast area.

Breast implant removal surgery can address a variety of concerns, including: capsular contracture, implant malfunction and dissatisfaction with breast size. If a woman chooses not to replace the breast implants, a breast lift may be required to address the skin that has been stretched.

With breast implant surgery, a revision or replacement surgery is usually required within 10–15 years.

In some cases, breast implant removal and/or replacement procedures need to be performed in two stages. The first stage is the removal of the implants and capsulectomy. The second stage is the insertion of new implants and/or breast lift.

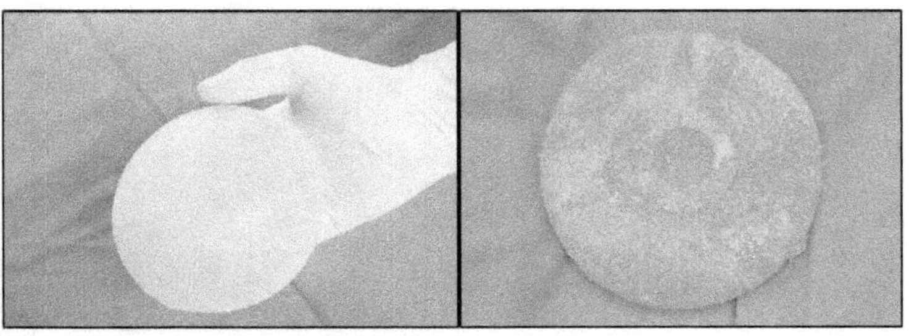

New breast implant   Explanted old implant

1.4 Breast Implants Associated Anaplastic Large Cell Lymphoma (BIA-ALCL)

This is a rare and highly treatable type of lymphoma that can develop around breast implants. BIA-ALCL occurs most frequently in patients who have breast implants with highly textured surfaces. This is a cancer of the immune system, not a type of breast cancer. When caught early, BIA-ALCL is usually fully curable by removing the implants and the capsule. It takes an average of seven-to-ten years after implant insertion before the lymphoma develops.

The most typical presentation is a fluid swelling around the breast implant and in the space between the implant and breast implant capsule.

In 2019, the Australian Therapeutic Goods Association (TGA) announced that it was considering regulatory action regarding breast implants. This included suspending and recalling certain types of breast implants following an extensive review of an apparent association between Anaplastic Large Cell Lymphoma and some implants.

Anyone with breast implants needs to ensure they have their implants checked regularly by their specialist plastic surgeon.

While the majority of the implants are safe, and many women live full and rewarding lives with implants, the impact of Breast Implant Associated Anaplastic Large Cell Lymphoma (BIA-ALCL) is noticeable.

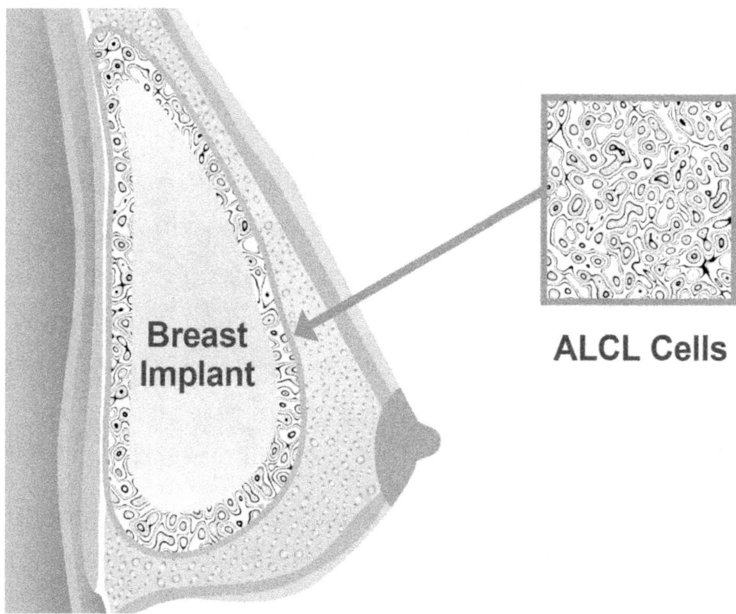

There are around 35 million women (60 million implants) in the world with textured breast implants. As of January 4, 2021 (ABDR, 2021), there were over 900 confirmed cases of Breast Implants Associated Anaplastic Large Cell Lymphoma (BIA-ALCL) worldwide and 123 cases in Australia. There have been over 32 deaths from late diagnosis of the disease worldwide, including four in Australia (Lonescu et al, 2021[1]). Estimates of risk and incidence have increased significantly recently, reaching 1 in 2,969 women with breast implants, and 1 in 355 patients with textured implants after breast reconstruction, based upon current confirmed cases and implant sales data over the past two decades. The incidence of BIA-ALCL cases in Australia is higher than expected, based on the population. About 1 in 7 of all cases reported globally are Australian cases.

1. Lonescue P. et al. New Data on the Epidemiology of Breast Implant-Associated Anaplastic Large Cell Lymphoma. *European Journal of Breast Health* 2021 (Oct); 17(4): 302–307.

However, it is important to put things into perspective by stating that the incidence of breast cancer among women who do not have breast implants is one in eight. Therefore, the incidence of BIA-ALCL is considered to be rare.

A unifying theory has been proposed by the authors of a paper in an epidemiology journal. The authors believe that the four factors likely to cause BIA-ALCL are:

1. Use of textured implants (with a higher risk for high surface area textured implants);

2. Bacterial contamination at the time of surgery to reach a threshold to cause inflammation;

3. A patient's genetic predisposition. The incidence of BIA-ALCL is lower in Asian populations;

4. Time for the process to develop, which is usually a seven-ten-year incubation period.

I recommend following strict protocols to minimise bacterial contamination. See the 20 points under the heading, "Safe Breast Implants Surgery Technique", earlier in this chapter.

These 20 points include: scrubbing the skin with Betadine; the use of a protective sleeve or delivery system; intravenous (IV) antibiotics; changing gloves frequently; the use of "No Touch" techniques; washing the pocket with saline; minimising the time of exposure; the use of techniques to minimise tissue injuries; careful haemostasis (to avoid bleeding); layered closure; and careful atraumatic dissection to reduce the risk of devascularised tissue.

I am proud to report that our clinics in Sydney have never had a reported case of Breast Implants Associated Anaplastic Large Cell Lymphoma.

CHAPTER TWO

Breast Lift

The breast lift, or mastopexy, is one of my most frequently requested plastic surgery procedures. Breast droop is common due to weight fluctuation, hormonal changes, pregnancy or breastfeeding. Sometimes women desire a breast lift because they wish to improve on their natural breast shape.

Breast droop following pregnancy can be caused by a hormonal softening of the ligaments that hold the breasts up and by tissue stretching. Changes in breast size during and after pregnancy can sometimes be quite dramatic. This is often accompanied by a loss of breast tissue, which means the breasts appear to sag and the upper half of the breasts look flat.

Minor degrees of breast droop can be effectively corrected by breast augmentation alone but, if the nipple is at or below the level of the breast crease, a breast lift will be required to recreate youthful looking breasts with high nipples.

A breast lift is often combined with breast augmentation if an increase in breast tissue is also required to restore the breasts to their former fullness, shape and position. Many patients who complain of breast sagginess, or breast ptosis as it is known in medical terms, will respond well to surgical lifting of the breast tissue, known as a breast lift or mastopexy.

Natural-looking breasts are the ultimate goal of breast enhancement surgery. This can be achieved through careful planning, a comprehensive breast examination and analysis. This includes precise breast measurements and a detailed discussion with the patient.

An implant trial will be performed to decide on the most appropriate size of the breast implants. Breast augmentation can be performed by fat injection using the patient's own fatty tissue or with breast implants.

The breast lift procedure creates a fine scar on top of the areola only (mini-lift), or a lollipop scar around the areola and vertically down (short scar breast lift) or a lollipop and a horizontal component in the breast crease (inverted T, a full breast lift).

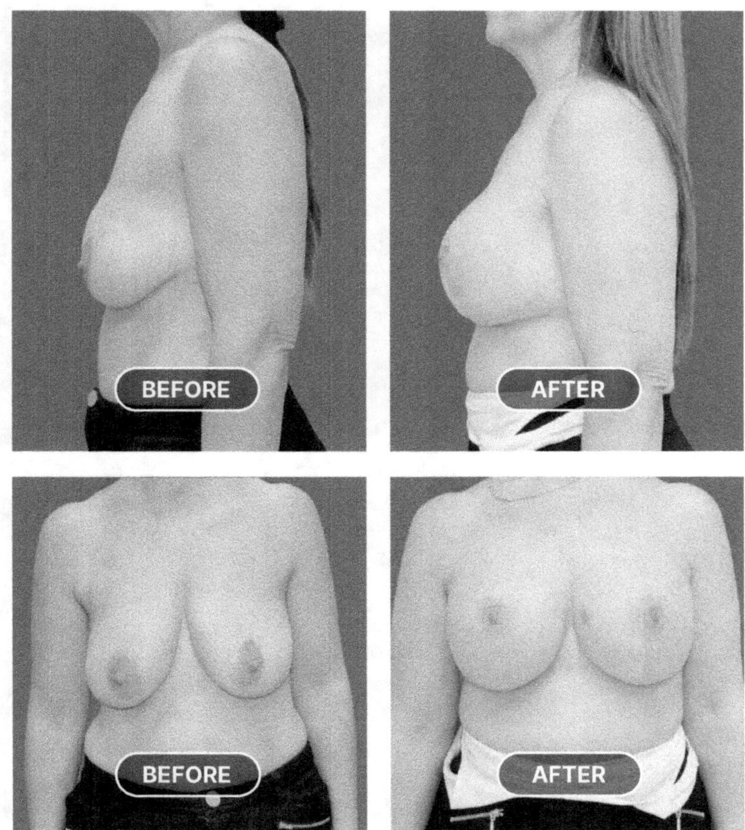

Breast lift and augmentation surgery using 375 cc round highly cohesive implants. The surgery included repositioning the nipples as they were previously below the level of the breast crease.

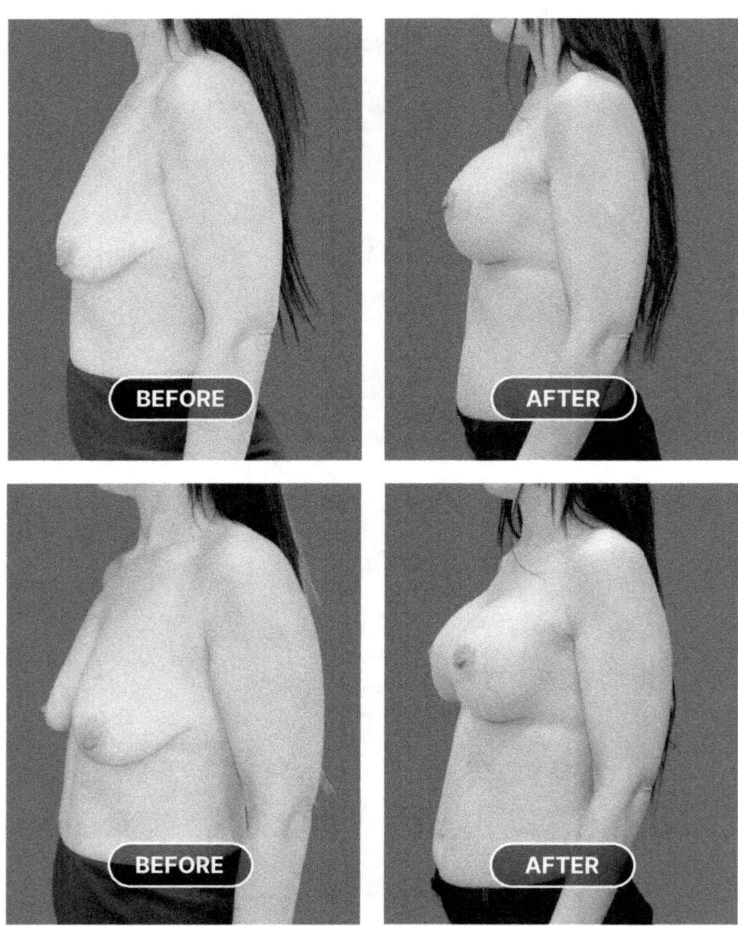

Breast lift and breast augmentation surgery using 375 cc round highly cohesive implants. The surgery included repositioning the nipples so that they are above the level of the breast crease. Before surgery, this woman had Grade II ptosis and her breasts lacked shape and volume.

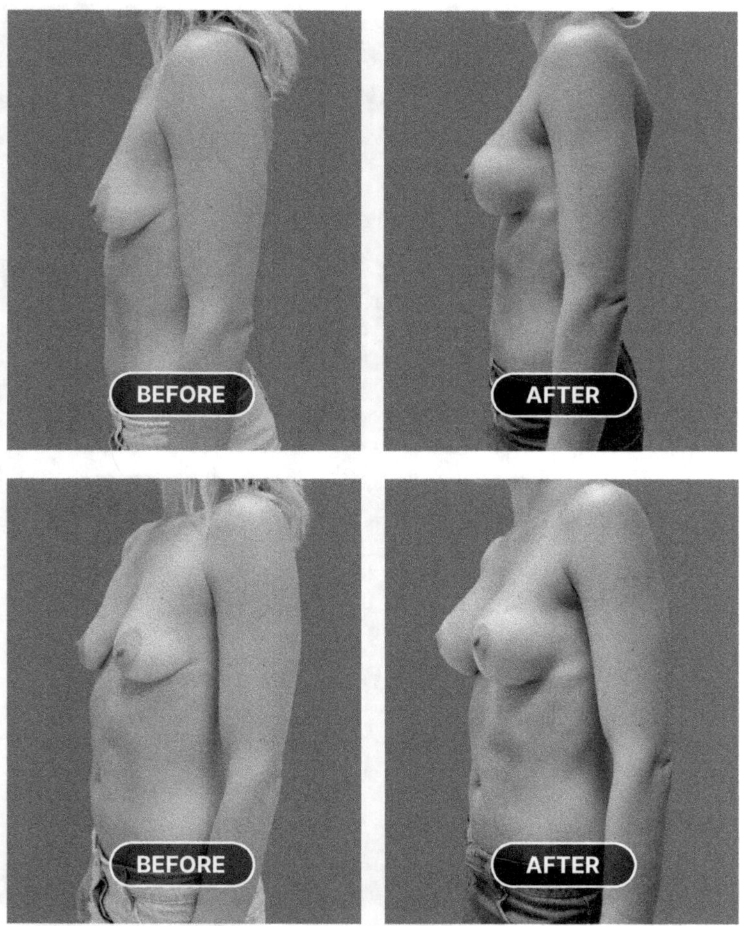

Breast lift and augmentation using 260 cc round silicone implants. This patient's areolae were reduced and the nipples lifted. Her breasts have been restored so that they are in proportion to her body frame.

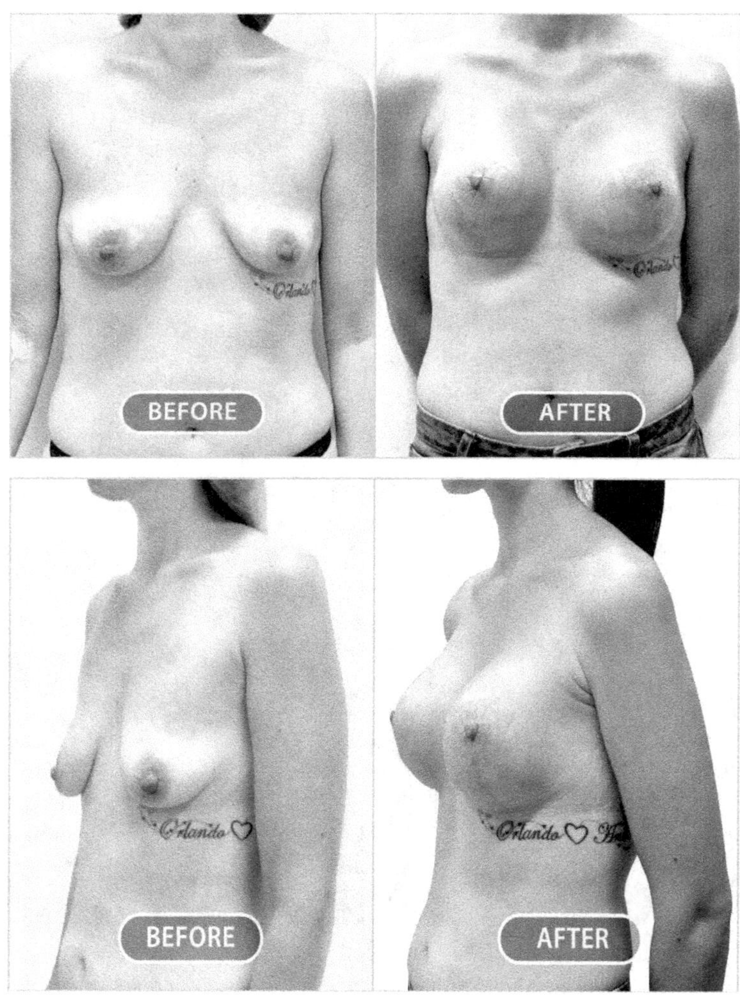

Many women choose to have a breast lift due to breast droop, caused by weight fluctuation, hormonal changes, pregnancy and/or breastfeeding. Note the proportionate breasts and higher nipples.

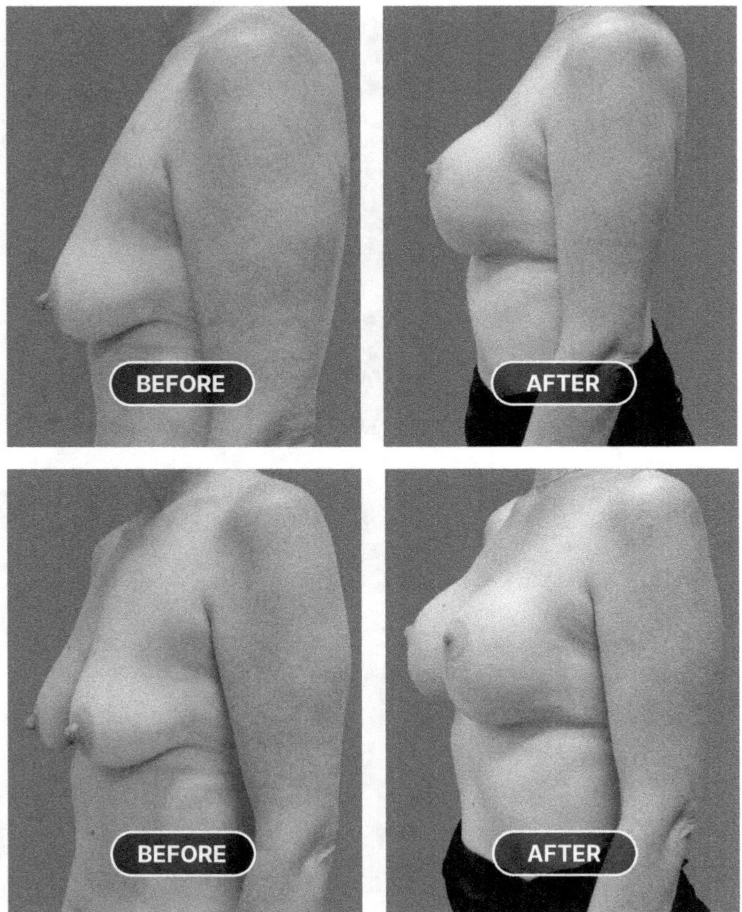

Breast lift and augmentation using 385 cc round implants to restore sagging breasts to a firmer, more pleasing shape. The nipples have been lifted and reduced in size.

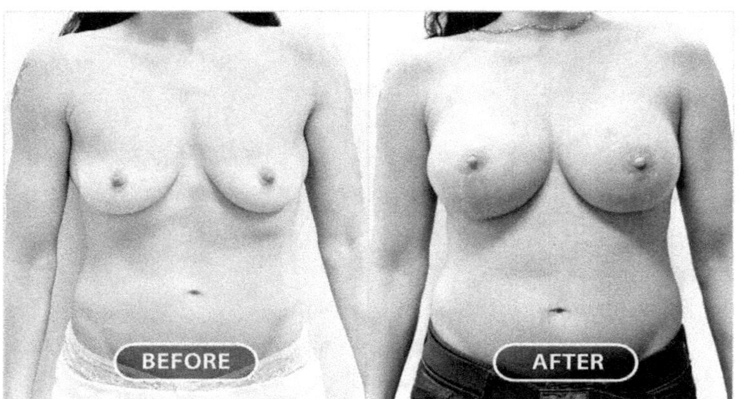

Breast lift and augmentation surgery. Note the sharp cleavage and proportionate breasts.

CHAPTER THREE

Breast Reduction

Large breasts may interfere with daily activities, such as sports. You may enjoy jogging, playing tennis and volleyball but have always had to wear two compression bras for support. Heavy breasts will eventually cause the formation of deep grooves on the shoulders from the weight of the breast tissue supported only by narrow bra straps.

Pregnancies, weight fluctuation and genetics are the main contributors to large breasts. They not only become heavy, but begin to sag as well as causing neck, shoulder and lower back pain. Overly large breasts also appear disproportionate to a woman's hips and the rest of her body.

Breast reduction surgery is normally performed under general anesthesia as day surgery or as an overnight stay. The procedure takes two-to-four hours to perform, depending on the size of the breasts and the amount of reduction required.

Breast reduction is a very satisfying procedure for patients, as it improves their posture, takes the pressure off their neck and shoulders as well as giving them better quality of life.

A combination of breast reduction and breast lift surgery produces healthier and lighter breasts. Lateral chest liposuction is a good adjunct procedure performed with breast reduction surgery to further define the outer border of the breasts and make arm movement easier and closer to the body.

My patients often report feeling immediate relief when they wake up from surgery to remove excess breast tissue. The breast tissue is sent for histological examination in a laboratory and is examined for any abnormal cells.

Note: For a discussion of male breast reduction ("man boobs"), please see Chapter 6: Plastic Surgery for Men in Dr Laith Barnouti's first book, *Your Guide to Modern Plastic Surgery*.

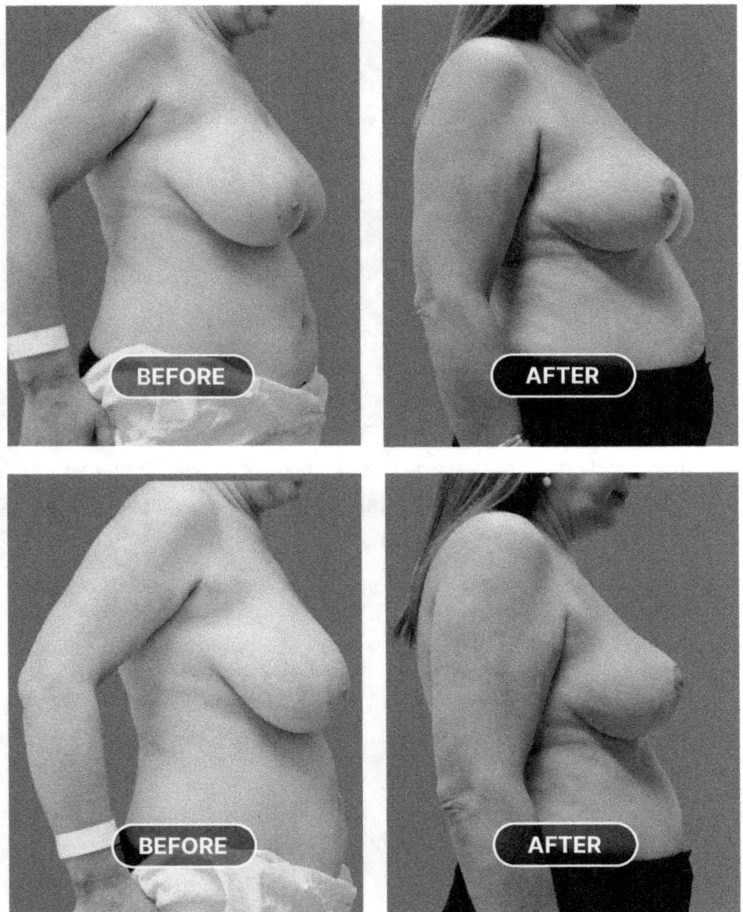

During this woman's breast reduction surgery, approximately 650 grams of breast tissue was removed from each breast, and she is now two cup sizes smaller. This patient's quality of life was greatly improved as her back pain diminished. She also has a better breast shape, and the nipple/areolar complex has been lifted.

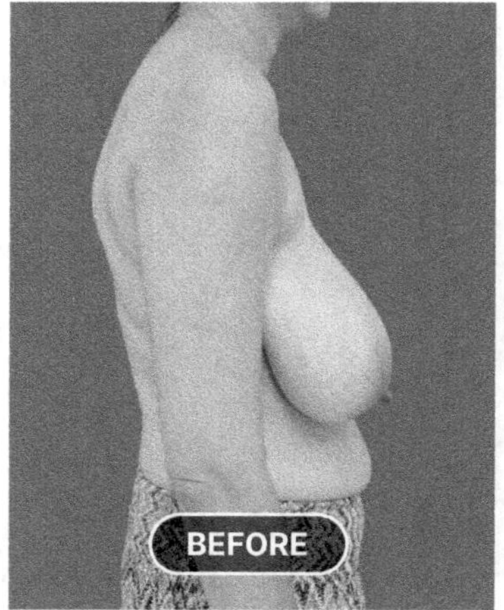
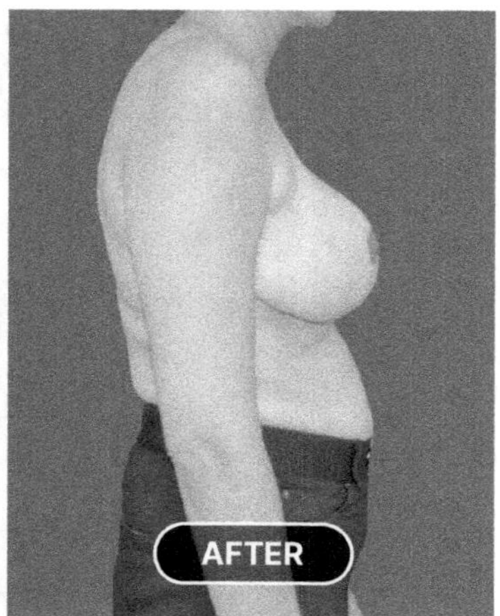

When a patient has to deal with a large breast size and disproportion, the body must constantly compensate, which overtaxes muscles in the shoulders and back, causing prolonged or increasing pain.

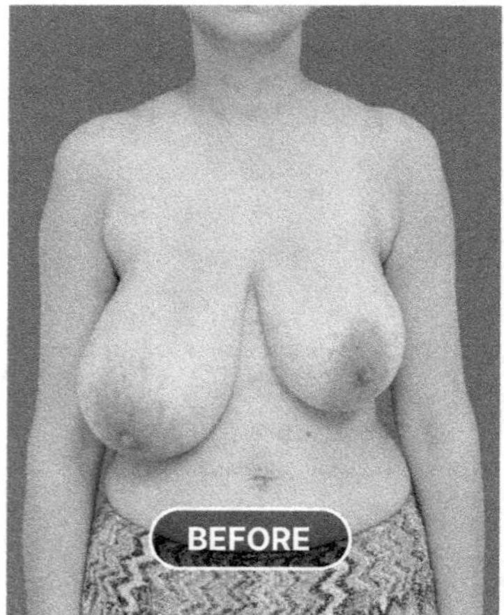
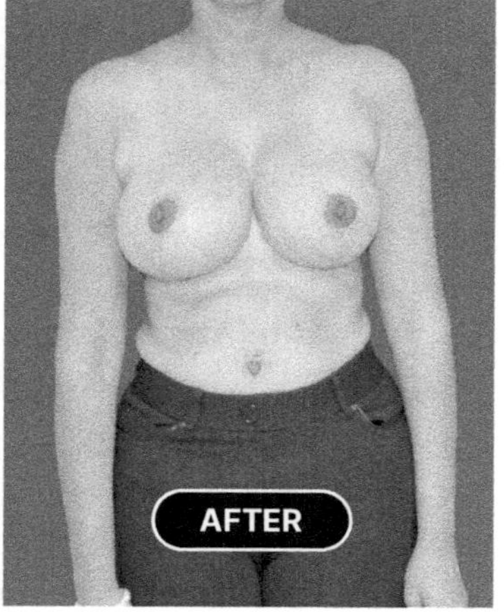

This woman suffered from congenital breast asymmetry exacerbated by weight fluctuations. Breast tissue symmetry was achieved by a breast reduction and higher lift on the right side and then augmentation with 375 cc round submuscular implants on both sides. Only experts should attempt this complex surgery as a single surgical procedure. The final outcome is improved breast shape, volume and symmetry.

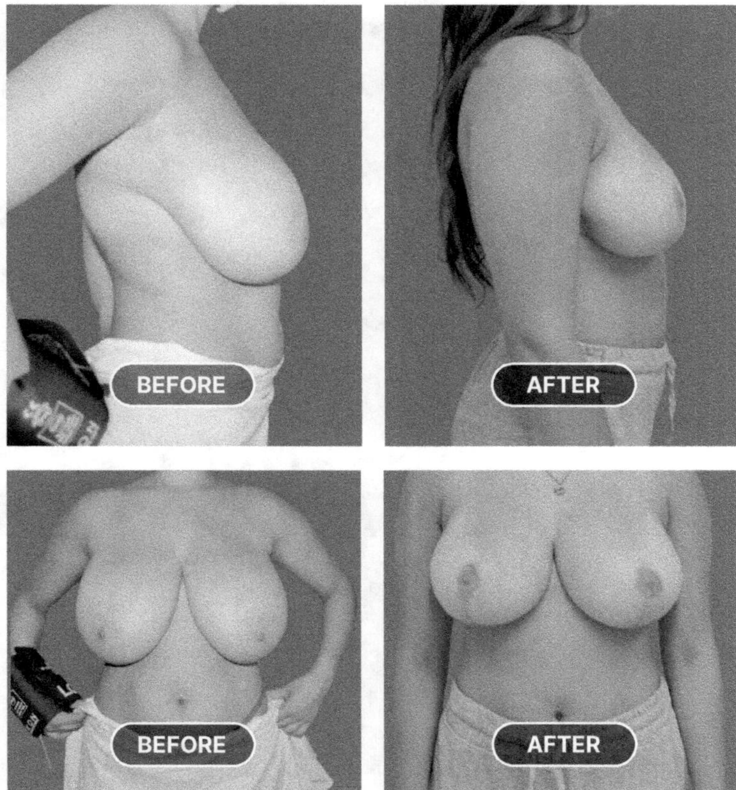

Breast reduction and breast lift. The patient now has smaller breasts and better shape in proportion to her body habitus. The red scar is still maturing. It can take up to 12 months for the scar to fade to a fine white line.

CHAPTER FOUR

Other Breast Surgery Procedures

4.1 Areola Reduction

Areolas are the pigmented part of the breast skin. When areolas appear disproportionately large due to genetics, pregnancy or heavy breasts, they can be resized and reshaped with an areola reduction procedure.

A wide areola diameter can be reduced to suit the rest of the breast tissue as well as the woman's nipple size and shape.

This 45–60 minute procedure is usually performed as day surgery. It can be performed alone or in combination with breast augmentation or breast lift surgery.

4.2 Inverted Nipples Correction

Inverted nipples can be classified as mild, moderate or severe based on the retractability of the nipple on manual stretching. This condition can be fixed through a simple surgical procedure.

This one-hour procedure is done under local anaesthesia, which makes the nipple area numb. It is performed through a small incision with literally no visible scarring and minimal downtime.

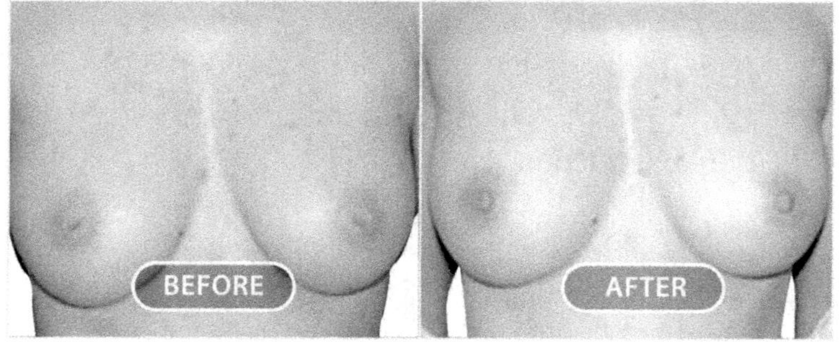

An inverted nipple repair may be done for several reasons.

4.3 Nipple Reduction

Nipples that are large (due to genetics or breastfeeding) can be resized and reshaped, making them more natural looking and less aged in appearance. Nipple reduction can be performed alone or in combination with breast augmentation or breast lift. This 30-minute procedure is completed through a small incision and leaves virtually no scars.

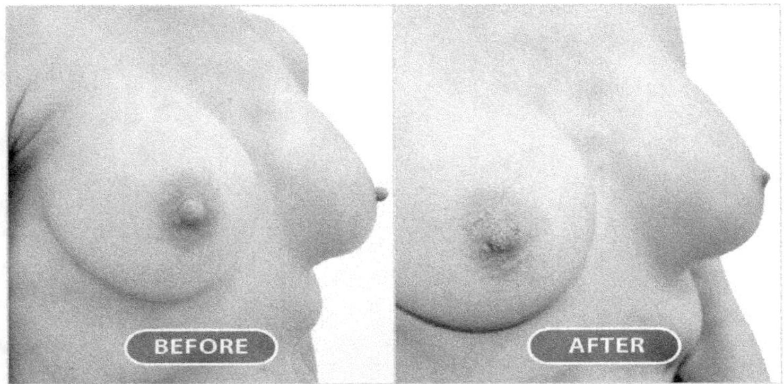

Before and after nipple reduction.

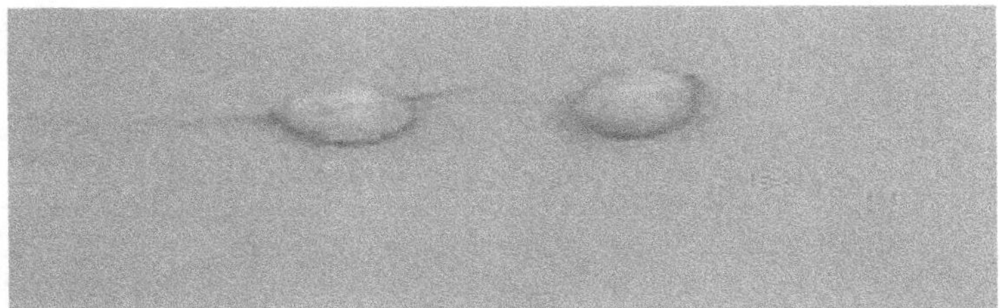

Amputated nipples

CHAPTER FIVE

Post Pregnancy Body Restorative Surgery ('Mummy Makeover')

Although having children is one of life's greatest gifts, pregnancy, childbirth and breastfeeding can take a huge, and often irreversible, toll on a woman's body. It leaves many mothers frustrated and dissatisfied with their appearance.

With our fun-loving beach culture, Australian mothers are usually keen to maintain their figures and body confidence. But after having a baby, some parts of their bodies will never return to their original shape or condition, no matter how much weight they lose or how much exercise and toning they do.

A Mummy Makeover is a combination of several plastic surgery procedures, which are custom designed for each woman to achieve the desired results.

The procedure is popular with women in their twenties, thirties and forties; in particular for women who have finished having babies and want to reclaim their body.

The Mummy Makeover includes some or all of the following plastic surgery procedures:

- Tummy tuck (also known as abdominoplasty);

- Pubic lift and mons pubis reduction;

- Liposuction to the tummy, hips, flanks and thighs;

- Breast enlargement, breast lift (with or without implants) or breast reduction; and

- Vaginal rejuvenation, including labiaplasty and/or pelvic floor muscle restorative surgery, also known as vaginoplasty.

Labiaplasty is a procedure that involves trimming the excess inner vaginal lips. Vaginoplasty is performed to narrow and restore the vaginal muscle to pre-childbirth status. Vaginoplasty helps prevent uterine prolapse, increases friction during intercourse, as well as restoring sexual confidence and pleasure.

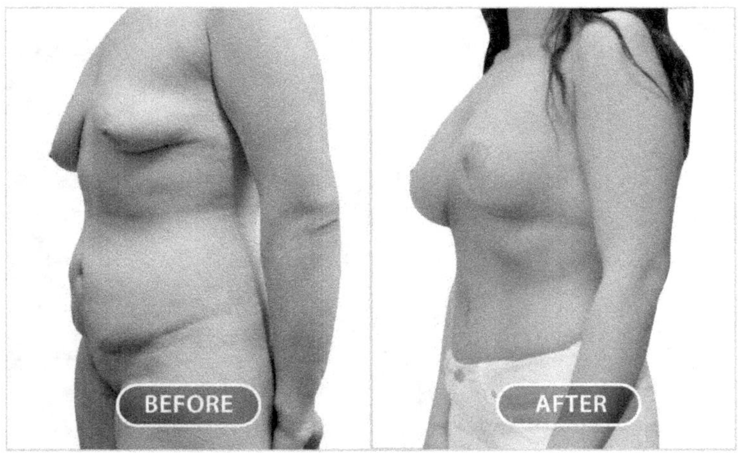

Mummy makeover: tummy tuck, liposuction and breast surgery.

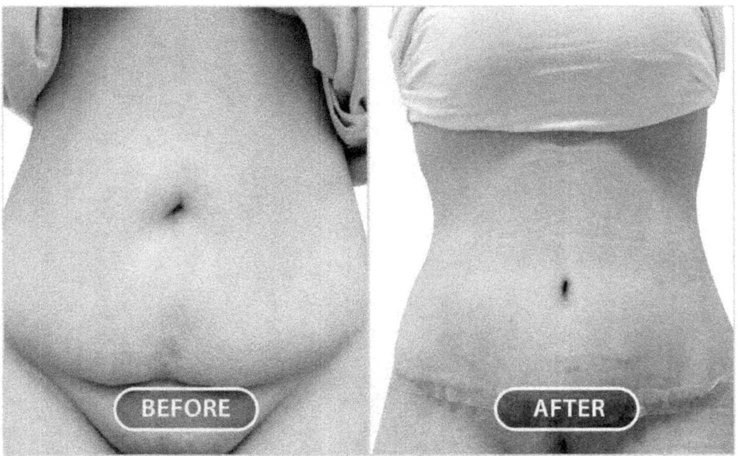

A large umbilicus is unattractive. Notice the small umbilicus in the after photo. The abdominal scar is positioned very low to reduce the mons pubis and lengthen the appearance of the torso. The use of liposculpture to produce an hour-glass figure is an important part of tummy tuck surgery.

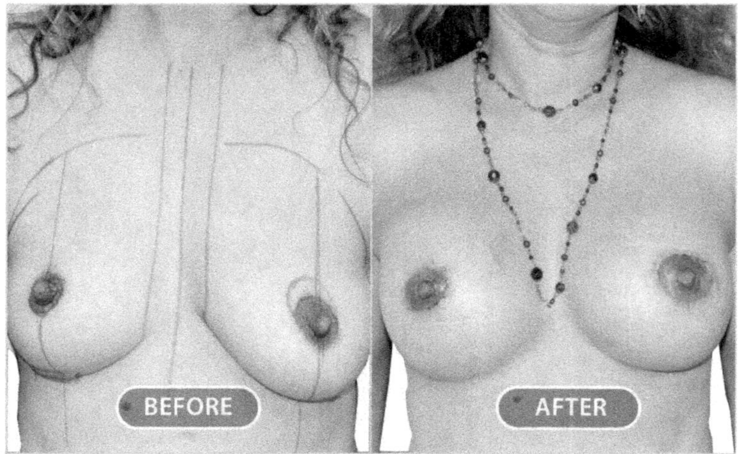

Breast augmentation through a small scar on the boarder of the areola.
The left side required a mini lift to achieve better symmetry.

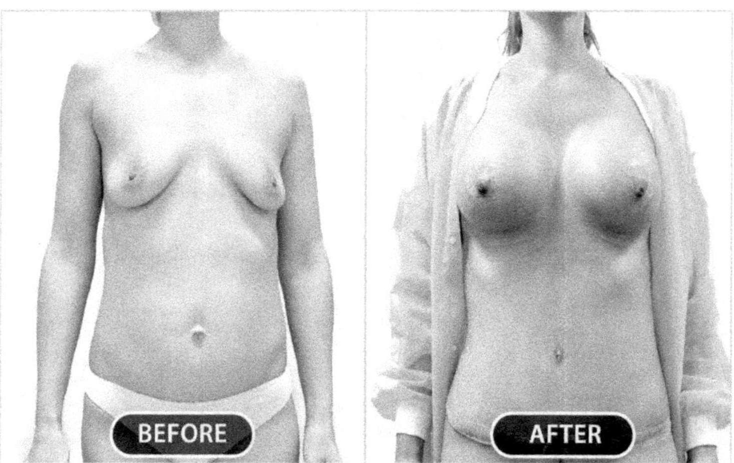

This patient had abdominoplasty, along with a breast lift and breast
augmentation. Attention to detail produces an artistic cosmetic abdominal
unit, a small umbilicus, a short mons pubis and low abdominal scar. Notice
the breast fullness and the nice cleavage in the after photo.

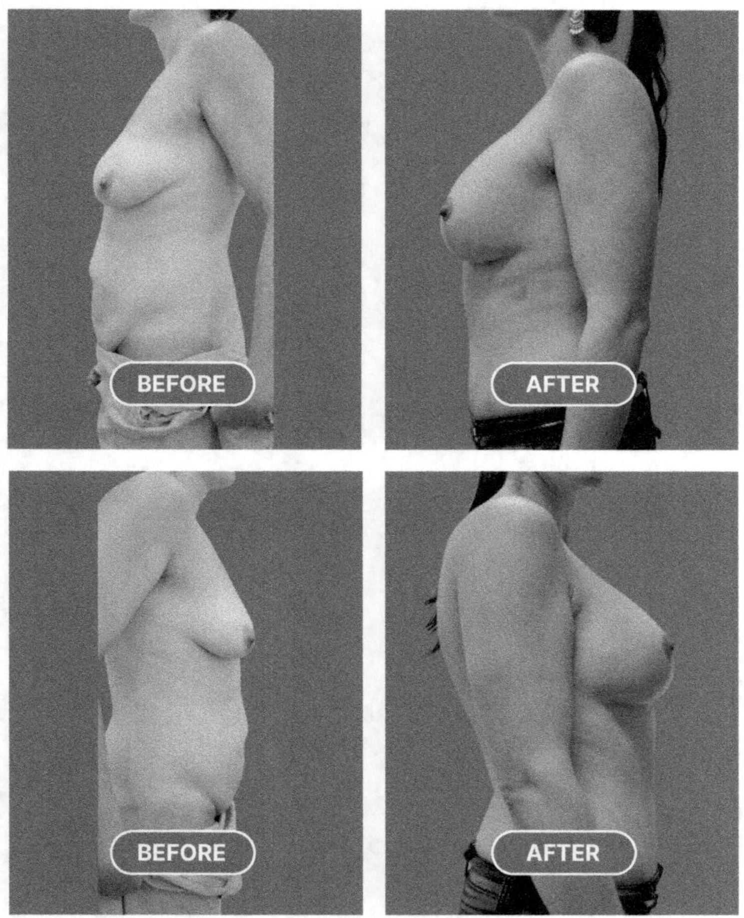

This patient had a breast lift, breast augmentation with 350cc highly cohesive silicone implants and abdominoplasty as part of her Mummy Makeover procedure.

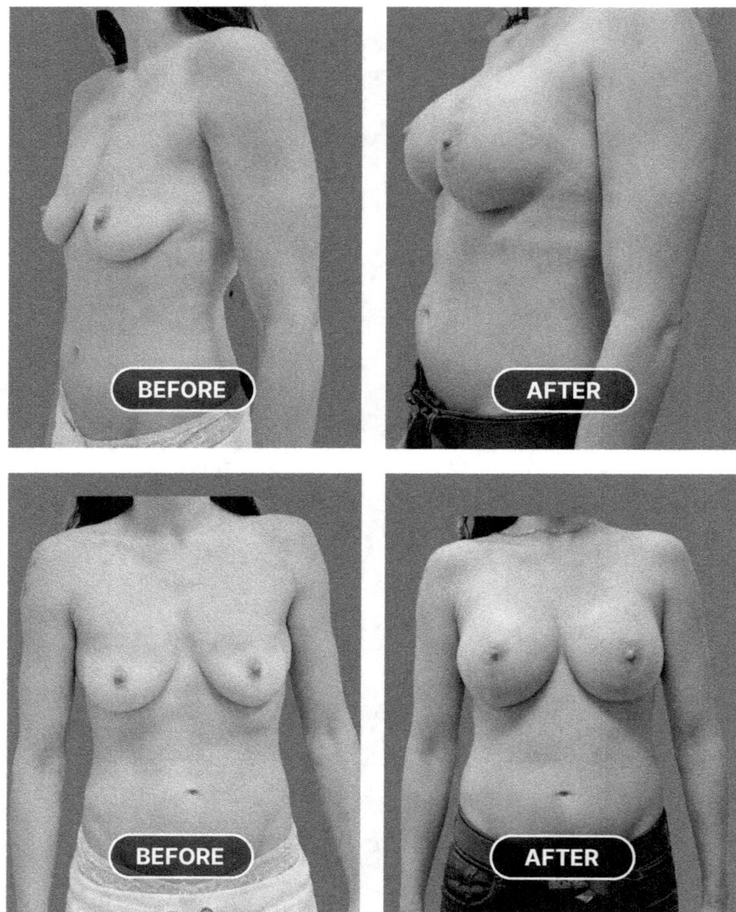

Post-pregnancy breast lift and breast augmentation using 420 cc round implants: dual submuscular pocket. Before surgery, the patient had a mild degree of sagginess and a slight natural asymmetry of her breasts. Patients are educated during the consultation about the fact that a slight natural difference between the two sides of the body is normal. Notice how the breast has been reshaped post surgery and the areolar/nipple complex lifted above the breast crease line.

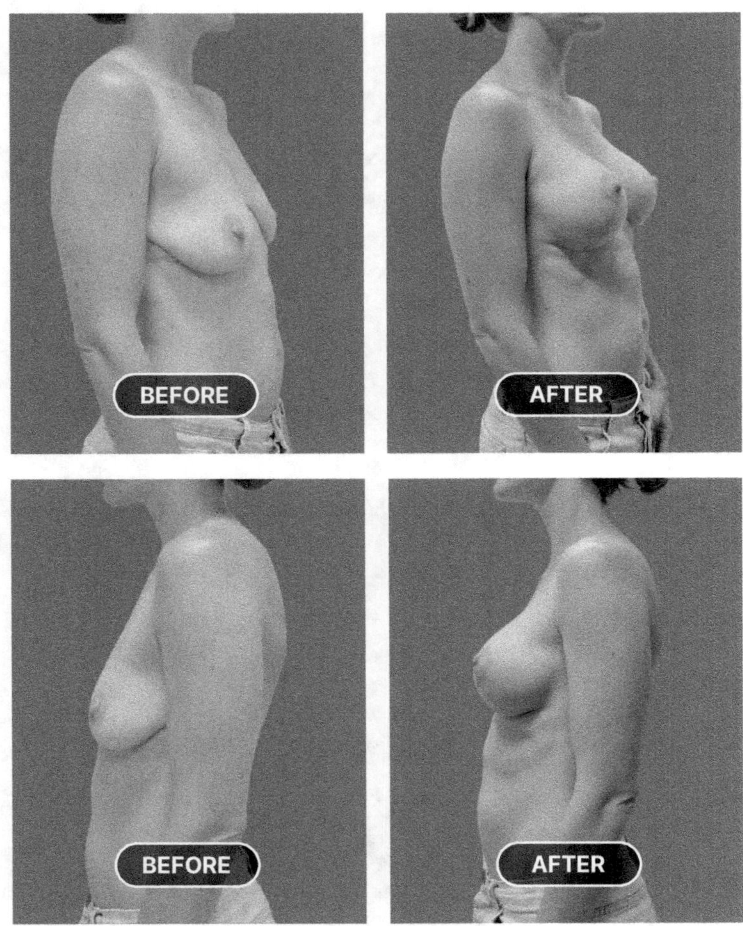

Some Mummy Makeovers include only breast surgery procedures. This woman had breast augmentation using 280 cc round high profile implants and a breast lift with a vertical scar – also known as a lollipop scar. The scar will mature and fade during the 12–18 months post surgery.

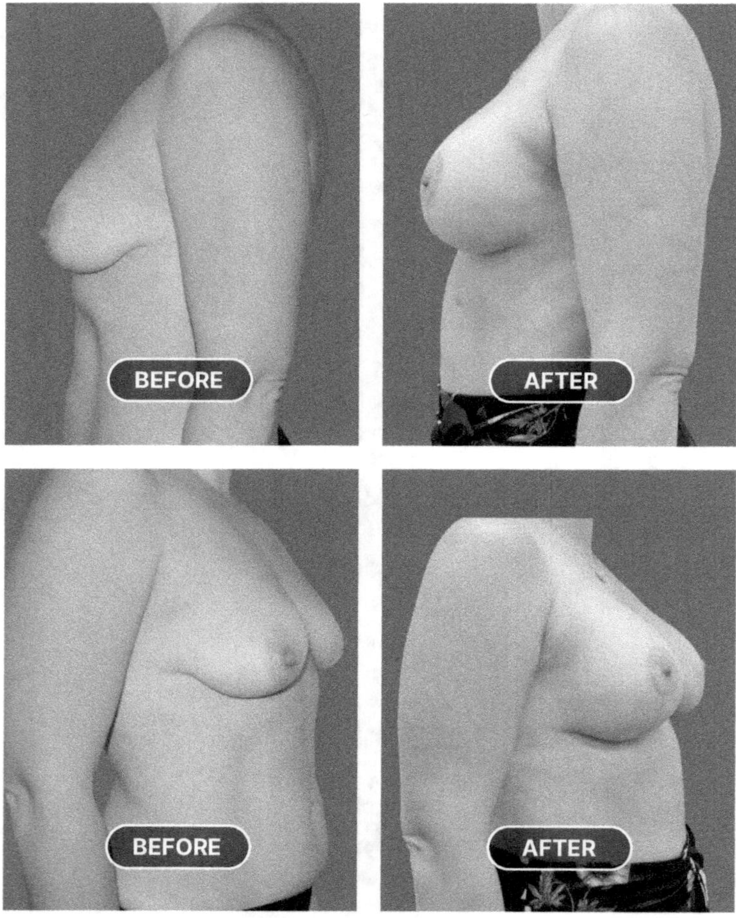

This woman had breast lift and breast augmentation surgery using 360cc round implants. Notice the recent lollipop scar. The redness of the scar will reduce to a fine white line as the scar matures.

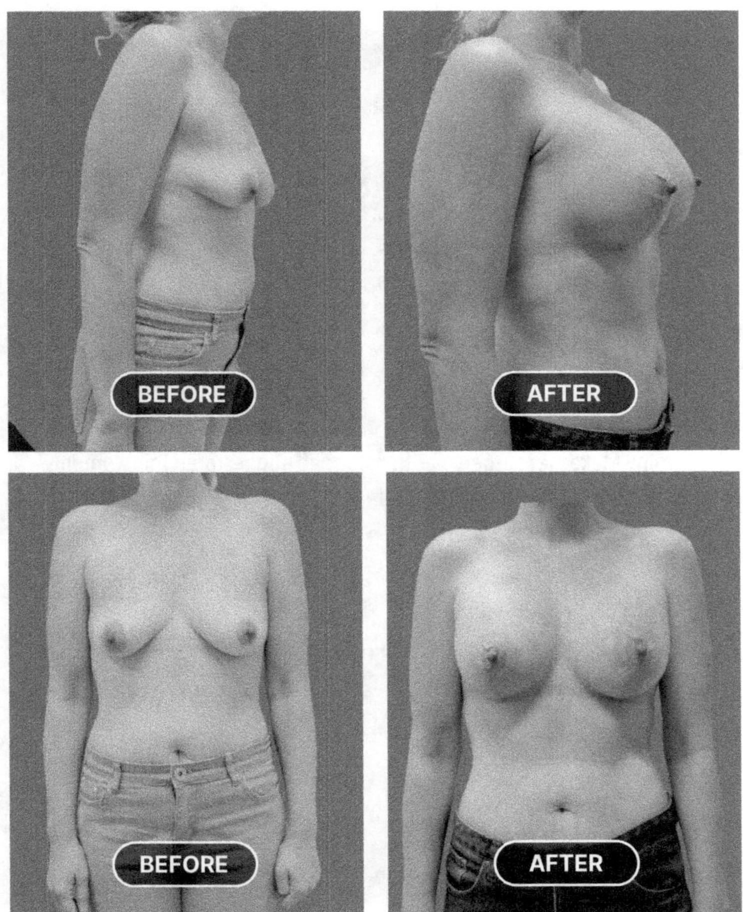

Breast lift and breast augmentation with 385 cc highly cohesive silicone implants. Notice the improved symmetry of the breasts and the higher position of the nipples.

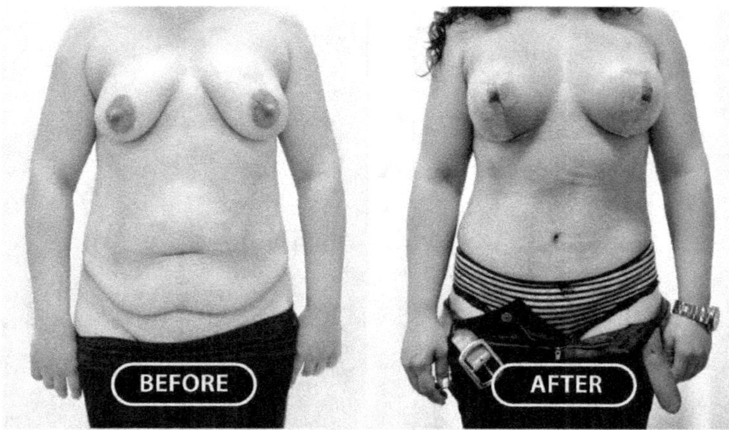

Mummy Makeover surgery has transformed and restored this women's body. When this surgical procedure is performed properly, it is done only once in a patient's lifetime.

CHAPTER SIX

Post Weight Loss Plastic Surgery

Many people who lose a significant amount of weight end up with excess skin that won't shrink back to its old dimensions. Others feel that certain body parts have succumbed to gravity and that they are slowly sliding to the floor. Where a facelift can give the impression of youth, it is only a partial remedy if other parts of your body tell a different story. Body makeovers are a "complete package" that restore a youthful look everywhere it's needed or desired.

Individuals who are overweight due to genetics, lifestyle habits or post-pregnancy, are willing to try anything to lose weight and get back into shape. A small percentage of them can achieve their goals through diet and exercise. An even higher percentage of people, however, find that their weight interferes with exercise and confounds the problem. They find themselves in a "Catch 22" situation; they can't exercise because of their weight, and they are unable to lose weight because they can't exercise.

One popular solution for individuals caught in this situation is to have bariatric surgery. This surgery is performed by a bariatric surgeon and is designed to modify the stomach and intestines so that weight loss is possible. Bariatric surgery has been very effective in producing significant weight loss for many people who feel they have no other option.

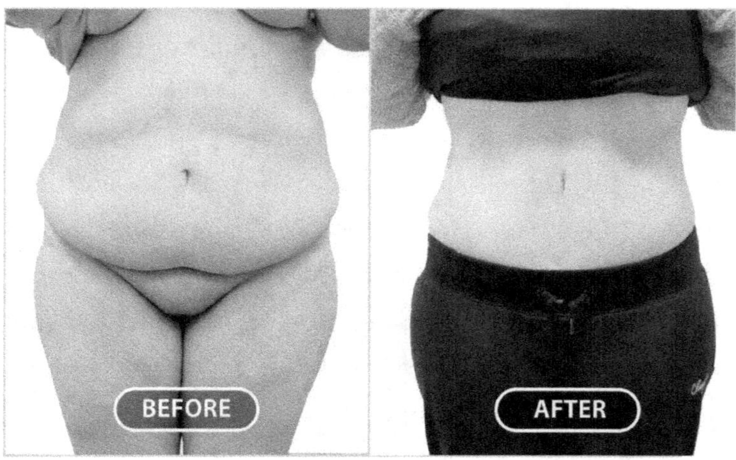

Excess skin removal is often necessary after excessive weight loss. A number of procedures were performed on this patient, including pubic lift, repaired muscle separation, and liposculpture.

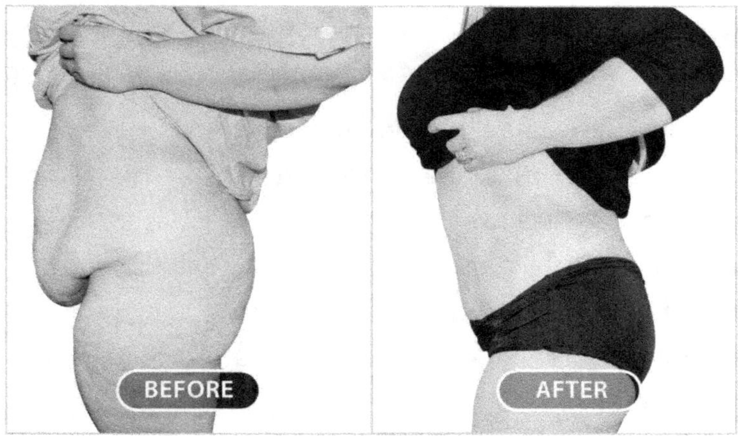

Post weight loss abdominoplasty.

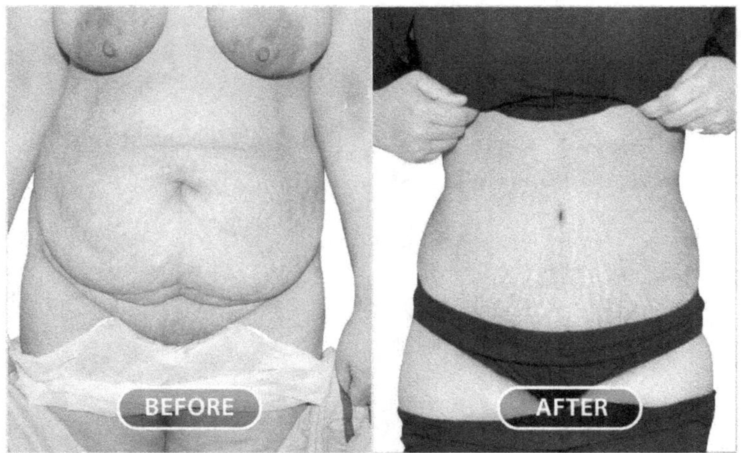

Extended radical abdominoplasty, liposculpture, pubic lift and umbilical reshaping.

Plastic surgery procedures following massive weight loss are generally extremely gratifying for both the patient and the surgeon. The outcomes are usually dramatic and offer a significant functional and aesthetic benefit to the patient.

These procedures address the loose skin that remains after the weight is gone. While someone is overweight, the skin stretches to accommodate the increased volume of fat. After weight loss, the skin often fails to tighten, and therefore it sags or even hangs. It acts as a continuous unattractive reminder of the person's previous weight and figure.

Unfortunately, diet and exercise will not tighten the skin (exercise never tightens skin, only muscles). The only way to tighten and/or remove loose skin is through surgery.

Depending on an individual's unique situation, there are a number of surgical options:

- A facelift to eliminate loose face and neck skin;

- A tummy tuck to eliminate loose abdominal skin;

- A pubic lift to eliminate the overhanging part of the mons pubis;

- An arm lift to eliminate loose arm skin;

- A breast lift to eliminate loose breast skin;

- An inner thigh lift to eliminate loose inner thigh skin; and

- A buttock lift to eliminate loose thigh and buttock skin.

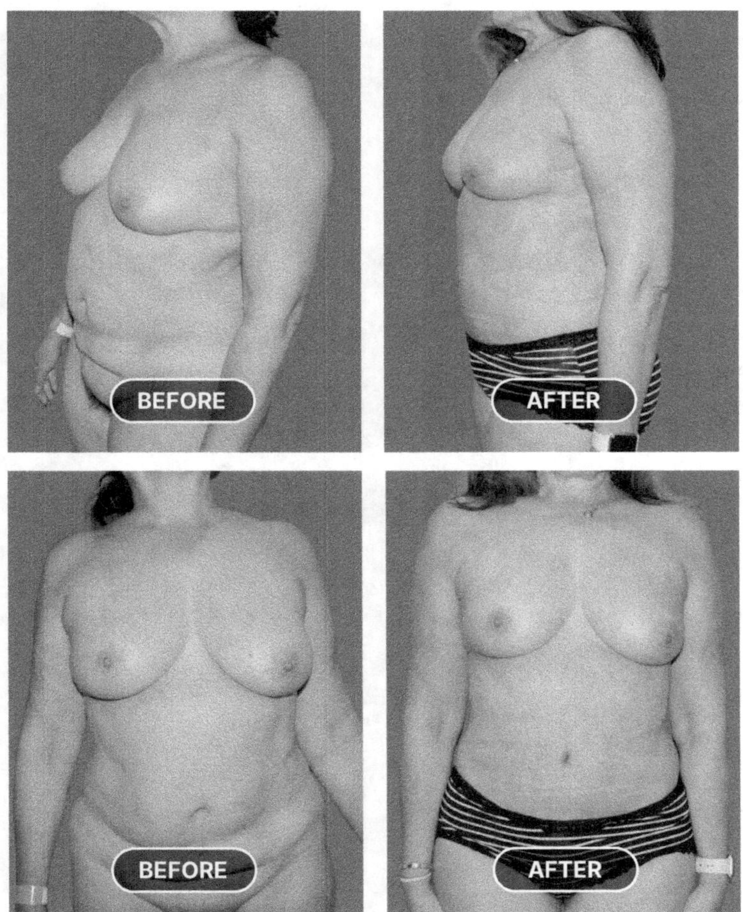

This patient underwent a tummy tuck and breast reduction by liposuction. When the breast tissue is of good quality and the nipples are not too low, then a breast tail and lateral chest liposuction helps to reduce the breast size. Notice the well-defined outer border of her breasts in the after photo. This definition was achieved by liposuction.

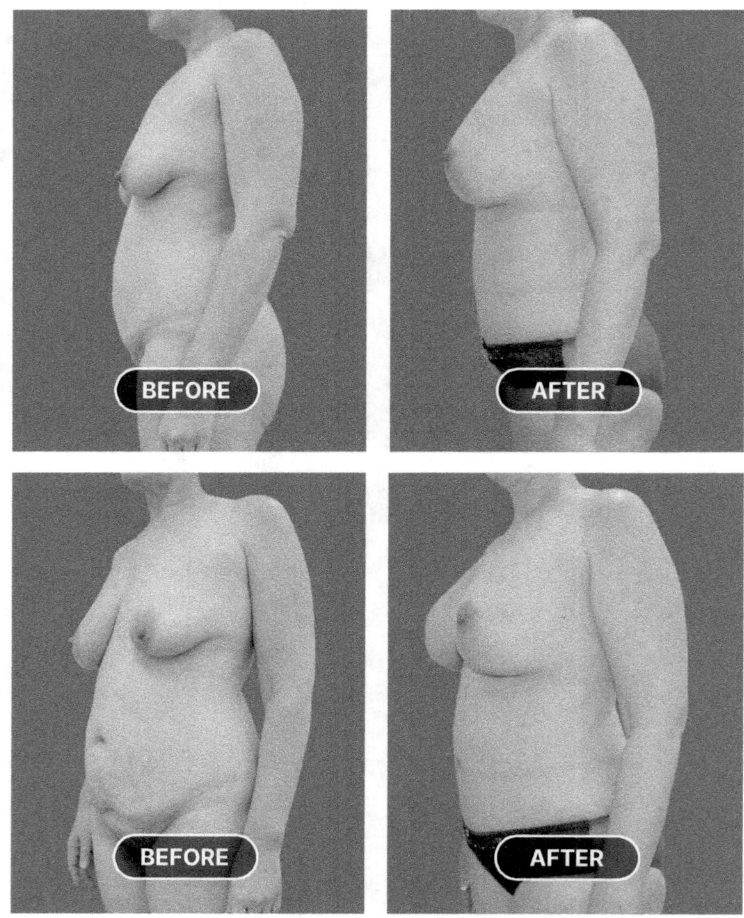

This patient had a tummy tuck, breast lift and breast augmentation surgery using 400 cc round submuscular implants. Notice the reshaped breasts and higher level of the nipple after surgery.

Most individuals who achieve significant weight loss will often require a few of the above operations. The surgery is tailored to fit the patient's needs, beginning with the area of highest concern. Most substantial weight loss patients prefer to start with a tummy tuck and breast lift, with or without breast enlargement, for shape enhancement.

The body lift is performed under general anaesthetic in a hospital and takes five-to-seven hours depending on its complexity. It must not be entered into lightly. As with any surgery, there will be scarring. The more skin that requires removal, the longer the scar. For a body lift, scars will range from along the lower abdomen, around the hips, and toward the buttock crease.

There is an additional scar in each groin crease due to the inner thigh lift. One way to look at it is that this operation exchanges one cosmetic problem (loose skin) for another (scars). Generally, those with very loose saggy skin following substantial weight loss are likely to find that this trade-off is worthwhile. Those with only a small amount of looseness will perhaps decide they do not want the scars.

CONCLUSION

As someone who keenly observes how humans age (myself included), I'm intrigued to learn about every method available that can safely and reliably help people maintain and improve their looks and body.

I love what I do and find it very satisfying to improve my patients' lives through plastic surgery. I'm passionate about safety as well as medical and surgical expertise. And, as my attention to detail will attest, I have developed a finely tuned eye for natural beauty.

It is my desire to soften the effects of ageing in my patients. Life is stressful enough as it is. If I can provide my patients with a more rested and happier look … If I can help them increase their satisfaction with their bodies and improve their quality of life … If I can help them achieve their goals when it comes to their appearance and physique, then I have done my job.

My final advice is not to rush into surgery, but instead take your time and think about what surgery can and cannot do for you. Planning for surgery is the most crucial part. Do not worry about the smallest details of techniques; that is the job of your plastic surgeon. Rather, prepare yourself for your recovery period, which may be unpleasant and take from two days to four weeks depending on the surgical procedure.

Also remember that you are doing the surgery for yourself – to improve your physical appearance and boost your confidence – not for others.

Good luck on your journey to a new you!

Dr Laith Barnouti

SPECIALIST PLASTIC SURGEON, FRACS
CONJOINT SENIOR LECTURER, THE UNIVERSITY OF NSW
SYDNEY, AUSTRALIA